Life After Hip Replacement

A Complete Guide to Recovery & Rehabilitation

Life After Hip Replacement

A Complete Guide to Recovery & Rehabilitation

by
Troy A. Miles, MD

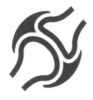

Stay active. Live healthy. Get inspired.

Sign up today to get exclusive access to the most authoritative, useful, and cutting-edge information for hip replacement, knee replacement, and shoulder replacement surgery.

Visit us online at www.reddinghipreplacement.com
Join our mailing list at www.reddinghipreplacement.com/join

This book is not a medical manual. The information given here is designed to help you make informed decisions about your health. It is not intended as a substitute for any treatment that you may have been prescribed by your doctor. If you suspect that you have a medical problem, we encourage you to seek competent medical help.

Mention of the specific companies, organizations, or authorities in this book does not imply endorsement by the author or the publisher.
Internet addresses given in this book were accurate at the time it went to print.

Project Credits
Editor: Stephanie Miles
Cover Design: George Ilian
Illustrations: Septiana Budyastuti

Manufactured in the United States of America

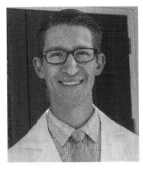 TROY A. MILES, MD is a practicing orthopaedic surgeon in Redding, California, who specializes in the treatment of disorders of the shoulder, hip, and knee, including joint replacement and reconstruction, and arthroscopic surgery. Dr. Miles is a member of the American Association of Hip and Knee Surgeons, American Orthopaedic Association, American Association of Orthopaedic Surgery, and the North Pacific Orthopaedic Society. He has lectured at the Annual Meeting of the North Pacific Orthopaedic Society, the Annual Meeting of the American Society of Surgery of the Hand, and the Annual Meeting of the American Association of Orthopaedic Surgery.

Dr. Miles maintains an active interest in academic medicine, as clinical faculty at UC Davis Medical Center in Sacramento, California.

Preface

For some, a pain-free life is only a memory. Thanks to advancements in the field of orthopaedic medicine, it doesn't have to be.

Through my experience as an orthopaedic surgeon who specializes in the treatment of disorders of the shoulder, hip, and knee, I have helped hundreds of men and women suffering from hip arthritis. It has been a privilege and a pleasure to help these patients re-learn the way their bodies were designed to move, and to resume the physical activities they once enjoyed.

As surgeons, we've been trained to focus on the finest details of medical procedures. But the majority of questions I'm asked by patients have to do with what they can expect life to be like after surgery is complete. Will they be able to walk up stairs? Can they play tennis? And most importantly, will they be able to keep up with energetic grandchildren? I am delighted to present my strategies for making the recovery process as smooth as possible.

Many physicians are now finding that patients who have clear understandings of what life will be like after surgery have the highest rates of satisfaction, and guides like this are an excellent starting point in the education process. For years, I have wished there was a book that I could provide to patients who are considering hip replacement surgery, with clear descriptions of what they can expect throughout the complete recovery and rehabilitation process.

Finally, it is here.

Troy A. Miles, MD

Contents

Important Note

The material presented in this guide was created to provide a review of information regarding hip replacement surgery. Every effort has been made to offer readers accurate, updated information. The contents of this guide have been compiled through professional research. However, medical professionals have varying opinions and new advances in orthopaedic medicine are made very quickly. As a result, some of the information in this guide may become outdated over time.

The publisher, author, and editors, as well as researchers quoted in this guide, cannot be held responsible for any error, omission, or dated material. Neither the author nor the editors make any warranty, expressed or implied, with respect to the material contained herein. The author assumes no responsibility for any outcome of applying the information in this guide.

If you have any questions concerning the application of the material described in this guide, please consult a qualified surgeon.

Section 1
Introduction

Welcome to Life After Hip Replacement: A Complete Guide to Recovery and Rehabilitation. If you are reading this, it means you have decided to undergo hip replacement surgery, or you are at least considering it. It's likely that hip pain has limited your everyday activities, which may be negatively impacting your general health and weight. It may also be affecting your mental well being, limiting your ability to get out and interact with others or enjoy the times when you do.

Luckily for you, hip replacement surgery is arguably the most successful surgery ever devised, and it has the potential to change your life for the positive. But before we get to that, there are some things that you should know.

A small disclaimer before we get too far into the details of your surgery day and the days, weeks, and months that will follow.

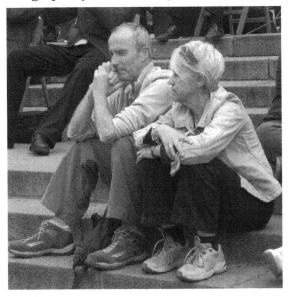

The decision to undergo total hip replacement surgery is one that should always be made in consultation with a licensed orthopaedic surgeon. This guide is intended to be a general overview of what life will be like following hip replacement. It should not replace the advice of your surgeon.

In addition to discussing your specific diagnosis, a qualified orthopaedic surgeon will be able to explain any non-operative treatment options for your condition, along with his or her approach to the treatment of disabling hip pain. No universal treatment will work for everyone, and undergoing hip replacement surgery is not a decision to be made lightly.

As hip pain is not a life threatening condition, and hip replacement surgery is an elective procedure, I always recommend that patients take their time and make sure that surgery is the right decision.

Making this decision requires an understanding of the process of recovery, rehabilitation, and the lifelong activity modifications that are necessary following a hip replacement procedure. The aim of this guide is to provide an overview of what to expect following surgery, including what to expect during your hospital stay and understanding which activities you should and should not participate in following hip replacement.

In this guide, we will not be discussing the details leading up to hip replacement surgery or the specifics of what takes place during the procedure.

My hope is that this guide serves as a springboard for the questions that patients ask their surgeons prior to having hip replacement surgery.

Specific advice regarding recovery, rehabilitation, and activity modifications following hip replacement are individualized based on each surgeon's training and personal protocols. Most joint replacement centers also have informational classes where this information can be reviewed.

In *Life After Hip Replacement: A Complete Guide to Recovery and Rehabilitation*, we will cover:

Preparing Your Home

Home environment is an extremely important part of recovery. I will offer tips on how to make your home environment safe and encouraging of healing. I will also review the importance of having adequate help at home during the critical early phase of recovery.

Surgery Day

What to expect on the day of your surgery will be largely based on your surgeon and hospital, as well as your specific diagnosis. However, I will walk you through a typical surgery day and point out certain precautions to keep in mind.

Recovery

Postoperative recovery happens in two phases: early and late recovery. Early recovery is the immediate postoperative period when the body is recovering and healing from the surgery itself. This includes pain control and other interventions for monitoring progress following surgery, which will be reviewed in this section. The first phase of recovery lasts until the six week follow up appointment, at which point healing is essentially complete and the second phase of recovery begins. The second phase of recovery includes increased physical therapy, strengthening, and endurance.

Rehabilitation

Rehabilitation is where the real work is done. Surgery is important, as is choosing the right surgeon, hospital, and therapist. However, none of these elements are more important than the work you put into rehab and therapy following hip replacement surgery. In this section, I will go over what to expect during a preoperative consultation with physical therapists, in-hospital exercises and expectations, and the decision of whether to return home or stay in a skilled nursing facility following surgery.

Sports & Exercise

Returning to everyday activities is high on most patients' wishlists. Specific techniques and strategies can help people who've undergone hip replacement surgery safely return to their favorite activities and recreational sports.

Maximizing Results

A number of the factors that have been shown to improve outcomes following hip replacement surgery are within your control. These include diet, exercise, and precautionary measures. In addition to reviewing these factors, I will discuss the scientific evidence behind them, and offer ways to maximize your chances of a success outcome following hip replacement surgery.

Activity Modifications

Hip replacement surgery was originally developed to treat elderly patients who had become incapacitated and were unable to walk without severe pain. With the overwhelming success of this procedure, however, the indications for surgery have been expanded and younger patients are now finding relief. The specific activity modifications recommended to you are likely to vary depending on factors such as your age, activity level prior to surgery, and the perspectives of your surgeon. In this section, I will outline these recommendations and discuss the reasoning behind them.

When thinking about your recovery and rehabilitation from major surgery, it is important to take the long view and keep realistic goals in mind. If you could not dunk a basketball before having surgery, having a hip replacement will not make this possible.

But having a clear, defined goal and a reasonable expectation of achieving it will help during the tough times of rehabilitation and provide you with the motivation to work hard to reach your destination.

Recovering from joint replacement takes six to 12 weeks of hard work, but this hard work can translate into upwards of 20 years of relief from joint pain. I like to remind all of my patients that they are not alone in this process. Surgeons, nurses, and physical therapists play an important role in encouraging and supporting patients throughout the recovery period.

Now that you've gotten an overview of what to expect in this guide, let's get started.

Preparing Your Home

Advanced planning is the key to having a safe and effective recovery following hip replacement surgery. This planning process should begin with preparing your home and environment well before the day of your surgery. I recommend taking a look around your home and making the necessary adjustments beforehand to make recovery as easy and safe as possible.

Entryways

The first area of trouble for many patients is the porch or entryway of their homes. Porch steps and elevated entryway thresholds can be difficult to modify, and most patients only navigate these areas a small number of times in the first few days following surgery. Because the front porch and entryway are not heavily trafficked areas, you will be better served by focusing your attention on the areas of your home that receive more regular use.

Having said that, there are simple things anyone can do to make a front porch and entryway easier to navigate during the time when they are recovering from hip replacement surgery. Handrails or thresholds should be tight and secure. I also recommend removing loose doormats.

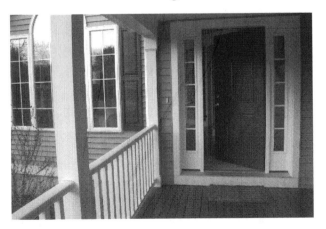

Depending on the time of year when your surgery takes place, yard debris, such as leaves or clippings, should be cleared.

Come up with a plan for who will take care of these issues prior to your surgery, since you will not be physically able to clear yard debris or make modifications to your home immediately following your procedure.

Main Living Areas

Inside the home, specific modification recommendations will depend on how your home is laid out and whether you have a single story home or a multi-level arrangement. Doormats should be removed, and shoes, umbrellas, briefcases, and any other loose impediments should be cleared and properly stored to decrease the risk of tripping and falling.

Establishing a recovery zone is one of the most important things you can do to ease the transition from hospital back to home. Your recovery zone should be an area with easy access to the majority of your immediate needs and wants, such as water, snacks, medications, a telephone, a television remote, reading materials, and games. It should also be close to a restroom and the space where you will be sleeping. Regardless of where you choose to establish your recovery zone, there are several steps you can take to make it safe. The first step is to remove loose rugs and electrical cords, as these are considered tripping hazards.

Coming up with the ideal seating arrangement following surgery can be a challenge for some patients, as well. I recommend making sure that your seating arrangement—the chair or couch where you will be spending the majority of your waking hours during the first phase of the recovery process—puts your hip in a safe position. What is considered a "safe position" will vary depending on the approach used by your surgeon. We will discuss this topic in greater detail later in this guide.

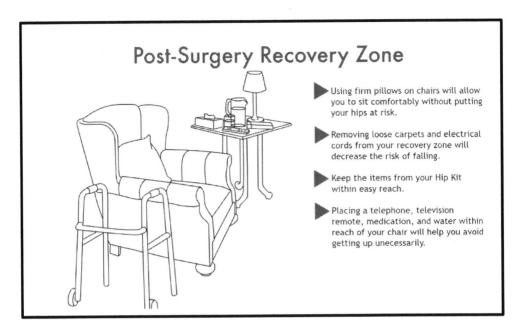

Post-Surgery Recovery Zone

▶ Using firm pillows on chairs will allow you to sit comfortably without putting your hips at risk.

▶ Removing loose carpets and electrical cords from your recovery zone will decrease the risk of falling.

▶ Keep the items from your Hip Kit within easy reach.

▶ Placing a telephone, television remote, medication, and water within reach of your chair will help you avoid getting up unecessarily.

The ideal seating arrangement involves a stable chair with a firm seat cushion, a firm back, and two arms. This arrangement allows your knees to remain lower than your hips, which minimizes the risk of hip dislocation. It is also important that you have firm pillows for any chairs, sofas, or car seats you may be using for the same reason. (This will be explained further in Section 4: Post-Operative Recovery.)

Couches are not ideal for patients recovering from hip replacement surgery, as they tend to allow you to "sink" into them. This flexes the hips excessively and makes it very difficult to get up from the couch safely. If you must sit on a couch, I recommend using a firm cushion or pillow to decrease this effect.

Sleeping Areas

Sleeping arrangements should be established well before coming home from surgery. In-home sleeping areas should not be more than a short distance away from the recovery zone. If you normally sleep upstairs, you may want to consider arranging a temporary place to sleep downstairs until you are able to comfortably navigate stairs.

Kitchens

The kitchen is another area of the home that contains a number of potential hazards for men and women recovering from hip replacement surgery. The same rules apply here as other areas when it comes to removing all loose impediments, such as rugs, mats, and cords.

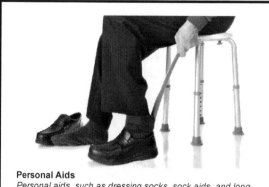

Personal Aids
Personal aids, such as dressing socks, sock aids, and long-handled shoe horns, can make it easier to get dressed and grab items around the house without losing correct body position. Reachers are another useful tool for picking up objects from the ground without excessively bending your hips.

It should be said that you shouldn't be spending significant amounts of time in the kitchen preparing food while you're recovering from surgery. This responsibility will fall on your caretaker, though you may want to make it easier on him or her by preparing meals beforehand that can be easily warmed and served.

Bathrooms

The next important area to focus on is the bathroom. Specifically, toilets and bathtubs/showers often need alterations for patients following surgery.

Toilets are quite possibly the most common source of hip dislocation during the early period following posterior approach hip replacement. Sitting on the toilet puts the hip in a very vulnerable position. To decrease this risk, there are a few simple modifications that patients can make.

One simple step, which everyone should complete prior to surgery, is installing a raised toilet seat.

Available by prescription or at any retail pharmacy, raised toilet seats substitute for standard toilet seats and help keep patients' knees below their hips. This prevents the body mechanics that can lead to hip dislocation.

Another toilet modification involves removing loose items from the back of the toilet tank. With those items removed, the back of the toilet tank can be used to support proper body positioning while sitting down and standing up. Removing any mats or rugs in the area, which could become tripping hazards, is also a smart idea.

A more involved measure for making the toilet safer after hip replacement surgery is to install permanent hand rails. While this endeavor may involve significant effort and cost, it also offers a more long-term benefit to patients. Once you have had hip replacement surgery, you will always have an increased risk for dislocation of the hip, compared to someone who has not had a hip replacement. Given that consideration, it may be worth investing in the installation of permanent hand rails alongside your toilet. This should be discussed with your surgeon.

The shower and bathtub areas should receive special attention to ensure safety, as well. Patients should not be taking baths until their surgeons have cleared them to do so. As a general rule, baths are not allowed until the wound is completely sealed and any remaining scabs have healed completely.

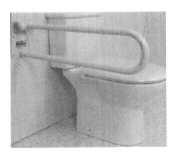

Bathroom modifications should be made before surgery takes place.
Hand rails or grab bars make it easier to use the restroom safely following surgery.

Several items can make showering safe after surgery:

1. *All patients should buy rubber non-slip mats, which help prevent slips and falls.*

2. *A secure safety rail for the shower can be invaluable. Installation of a permanent rail may be costly and may require significant effort, however there are several versions of temporary, stick-on rails that can be utilized during the early recovery period.*

3. *A stable shower chair or bench can be properly adjusted to maintain safe body position.*

4. *A handheld shower nozzle and long-handled scrub brush will help reach areas to be cleaned without significant alteration of body mechanics. This keeps the risk of dislocation as low as possible.*

One final word regarding bathtubs. If you have a bathtub that requires you to step inside, you will need assistance in order to enter and exit safely. There are many specific techniques for maintaining correct body position while entering and exiting a bathtub, and it is worth asking your physical therapist for guidance in these techniques.

Stairs

If you have a multi-level home, I recommend that you not use the stairs unless absolutely necessary. Even if you do not plan on climbing stairs, please take this opportunity to make your stairs as safe as possible. This means making sure that any broken stairs are repaired, that surfaces are not slippery, and that handrails are tight and securely fastened to the walls.

Several products are available, such as adhesive, non-skid stair covers, to prevent slipping. These can be found at most hardware stores.

Possibly the most important aspect of preparing your home for recovery from hip replacement surgery is arranging for in-home assistance.

Depending on your social situation, in-home assistance may come from a spouse, friend, or close relative. It is very important that you have someone with you in the first days after returning home from the hospital and that the person you select understands the responsibilities involved in this role. If you have a spouse who is not able to provide the level of assistance you will need, then you may need to arrange other forms of support, even if it requires that you have someone fly in to be with you during the recovery period.

Section 3
Surgery Day

What happens during a hip replacement surgery informs the recovery and rehabilitation process. Although this book is not meant to be a comprehensive guide to surgical approaches for hip replacement, it would be incomplete if I skipped over surgery day altogether.

In order for surgery day to run as smoothly as possible, I recommend arriving at the hospital approximately two hours before the scheduled start time. At that point, you will be checked in, prepped for surgery, and eventually taken to the operating room. Hip replacement surgery lasts between 60 and 90 minutes, after which time you will be brought to a recovery room. Expect to be under diligent observation for the next two hours, gradually becoming more awake, alert, and in a stable condition. At this point, you will be taken to your hospital room. Expect to work with a physical therapist for the first time on the same day as your surgery.

Some surgery centers are now offering same-day discharge for well-suited patients.

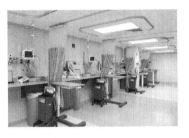

Expect to be checked in by several teams in the pre-operative area. You will be seen by your surgeon's team, the anesthesia team, and two nursing teams to ensure that you are ready for your operation and that there are no last minute issues.

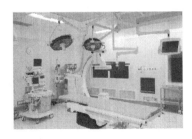

Once the check in process is complete, you will head to the OR. In the operating room, you will undergo anesthesia, have additional IV lines placed, and be positioned on the operating table for surgery.

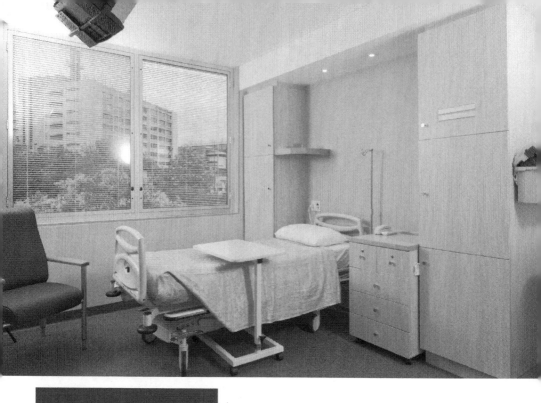

The early data on same-day discharge after total hip replacement seems positive, but for the purposes of this guide we will focus on the traditional inpatient setting for hip replacement surgery.

In order to make your surgery day as easy as possible, I recommend educating yourself about the process beforehand. Reading this book is a great place to begin, but it is not the only thing you can do. Ask your surgeon for a detailed guide, or even a pamphlet or printed handout, describing the specifics of his or her surgical protocols.

If your surgeon does not have a guide, there are several well-written guides available on the internet that describe what to expect on surgery day. Examples of these digital guides can be found in Section 11: Resources.

Make sure that all of your questions are answered prior to surgery day. Hopefully, the vast majority of your questions will be answered in this book and your surgeon's own guide. If they are not, then I recommend writing down your questions, so that you will not forget, and making sure that your questions are answered during the final pre-surgery appointment. The last thing you want while heading into surgery is to have anxiety because you don't know what to expect or your questions haven't been answered. An extensive list of questions to ask your surgeon can be found in Section 12: Frequently Asked Questions.

Post-Op Recovery

Postoperative recovery happens in two phases: the early postoperative period and the late postoperative period. The early postoperative period immediately follows surgery and lasts for the next six weeks. The late postoperative period picks up at the six week mark and typically lasts for an entire year. In this section, we will focus on the early postoperative period. Later, in Section 5: Extended Recovery, we will discuss the late postoperative period.

Early postoperative recovery from hip replacement truly begins in the recovery unit immediately following surgery. As was previously covered in Section 3: Surgery Day, once you have been taken to a hospital room and you are awake and stable, you will almost immediately begin working with physical therapy staff on early mobilization. At the very least, you can expect to be sitting on the edge of your bed, with the assistance of a nurse, within the first few hours following surgery. This early mobilization is important because it gets the process of recovery off to a good start. However, I advise patients that they should not do too much too early, as too much activity can set back the recovery process.

Doing too much too soon following hip replacement may increase inflammation and stress the tissues that were just operated on, making pain more difficult to control. This is an important concept to keep in mind throughout the early recovery phase.

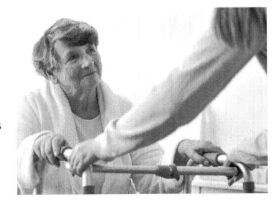

Even though you may feel good, and you may have the desire to do as much therapy as possible, pushing it too far immediately after surgery can result in unnecessary pain, and it will limit your ability to participate in therapy later during the recovery period.

Take the long view. The goal with hip replacement is years of function, and you won't achieve that in one day.

Listen to your body, take your time, and do what you feel comfortable with, but don't push too hard or you will wind up with a delayed recovery.

Physical Therapy

Physical therapy will typically begin on the first day after surgery. The extent to which you will mobilize will be based on how you feel and what you are able to tolerate. The goal here is to be able to safely get yourself in and out of bed and up to the restroom. Walking any distance on this first day after surgery is a bonus.

Expect to be uncomfortable on the day following your surgery. This will be one of the most uncomfortable days of the entire recovery period. The inflammation from your operation is peaking and the anesthesia from surgery is nearly completely worn off. As you begin to mobilize for therapy, these factors will combine and result in a painful hip. For this reason, there is a large focus on pain control by your care team on the first day following surgery.

Pain Control

Pain control is very important after total hip replacement. Again, without adequate pain control, a patient's ability to participate in therapy will be limited. Pain can also impact general health. Poor pain control may increase a patient's blood pressure, heart rate, and put his or her body in a state of stress.

On the flip side, too much pain medicine can also have serious consequences. Traditional pain medicine comes with numerous side effects ranging from simple annoyances, like itching and nausea, to fatal side effects, like breathing depression. For this reason, surgeons often try to only give patients the amount of pain medication they need — and nothing more. As surgeons, we also try to attack pain from different angles with multiple types of pain medications.

Pain control following hip replacement is an area of very active and extensive research. There has been a shift toward using a multimodal approach to postoperative pain control in the last decade. This includes different types of medications to address the different sources of pain, timing of medications, and specialized anesthesia techniques before, during, and after surgery for controlling pain and numbing the hip.

Surgeons can't take a one-size-fits-all approach to pain management because the pain that patients experience following total hip replacement comes from a number of different sources. During the first few days following surgery, pain may be caused by tissue

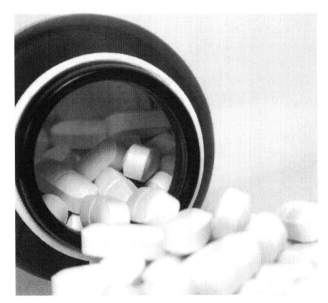

damage, inflammation, nerve irritation, and swelling, among other factors.

To address each of these sources, I recommend providing patients with medications aimed specifically at the source of pain.

A few examples of the different medication groups we have available are traditional opioid pain medications (such as oxycodone), anti-inflammatories (such as ketorolac), and nerve stabilizers (such as gabapentin). Surgeons may also recommend non-medicinal treatments like cold therapy, body positioning supports, and assistive devices to limit additional stress during the early phase of recovery.

Medication timing also plays an important role in helping to minimize pain following hip replacement. Pain control starts with pre-medication before surgery even begins. A pre-medication regimen may include all of the medications previously discussed in this section, along with special nerve blocks performed by an anesthesiologist before surgery begins.

Nerve blocks are injections of numbing medication directly targeting the nerves, which provide sensation to the areas in and around the hip joint. The idea behind this is that pain activates certain parts of the body's nervous system and brain, and if we can prevent these areas from being activated before a patient is in pain, then we can effectively decrease the overall level of discomfort after surgery.

Patients who have spinal blocks are able to participate in therapy sooner than those who receive general anesthesia. They also have fewer side effects, which may include constipation, nausea and vomiting, delirium, and low blood pressure.

A pre-surgery nerve block is followed by the spinal block for anesthesia during surgery. Spinal blocks have largely replaced general anesthesia for hip replacement because of the effects that general anesthesia can have on the heart, lungs, bowels, and mentation.

Avoiding general anesthesia has also been shown to decrease the rate of complications like heart and lung issues. (Horlocker et al. 2006)

Based on your specific health characteristics, along with the technical aspects of your surgery, you may be limited to just one type of anesthesia. The type of anesthesia you receive will be a decision made between you and your anesthesia doctor.

Pain control following hip replacement is an important aspect of recovery, but it can be challenging to manage pain for patients who have been taking opioid medications prior to surgery. Once the body has been exposed to pain medications, it develops a tolerance and more medication is needed in order to achieve the same level of pain control.

As you take more pain medication to control your discomfort after hip replacement surgery, the risk of serious complications continues to increase. For this reason, it is very important to work with your surgeon and the physician prescribing these medications to try and wean from the medications as much as possible leading up to surgery.

Your surgeon may also suggest that you see a pain medicine specialist to help in this weaning process. A pain medicine specialist may be able to recommend strategies for managing pain following surgery.

With all medications come side effects. Even if you receive a spinal block instead of general anesthesia, there is still a small chance that you may experience symptoms such as nausea, dizziness, and lightheadedness during your hospital stay. Nurses are trained to monitor patients closely, and these symptoms will be managed so you can participate fully in therapy and return home safely without delay.

The most consistent side effect of opioid pain medication is constipation. Inflammation from the surgery, the effects of anesthesia, and the relatively inactive state that patients find themselves in following surgery also play a role. To help decrease constipation, patients are typically given a combination of stool softening and bowel activating medications following surgery.

Based on your surgeon's protocol, there are several other medications that you may receive during your hospital stay. Please discuss these options with your surgeon.

Hospital Monitoring

While pain control is a large part of what your nurse and surgeon will monitor after hip replacement, there are several other aspects to recovery that are monitored closely, as well. One of these is breathing. As you will spend a large amount of time in bed, you will not be breathing deeply. When you are not taking deep breaths, this causes the small airways in the lungs to close, which creates the type of inflammation that leads to fevers. Fevers may occur in the first days following surgery, and they are something that nurses are trained to watch out for. Inflammation also increases the risk for pneumonia. To fight this, small breathing devices may be recommended to help you take long, deep breaths.

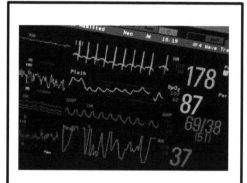

Vital Signs
Your vital signs (heart rate, breathing rate, blood pressure, and temperature) will be monitored approximately every four hours while you are in the hospital.

This can occasionally disrupt sleep, therapy, meals, and other activities, but is very important in ensuring continued health and well being during your hospital stay.

Vital signs can be monitored by a nursing assistant, your personal nurse, or if there are any concerns or issues, your surgeon. Occasionally, if other medical issues require more intensive care, an internal medicine doctor may care for you, as well.

Another area monitored by nurses and surgeons is the patient's ability to urinate. Medication, surgery, and immobility can prevent the bladder from working properly. The ability to urinate provides information regarding blood pressure and body fluid status. For these reasons, some surgeons elect to have a urinary catheter placed following hip replacement. However, this is an infection risk, and the goal is to get the catheter out as quickly as is safe. For this reason, some surgeons elect not to have a catheter placed following surgery. This is something to discuss with your personal surgeon prior to surgery day.

In many joint replacement centers, the majority of total hip replacement patients will go home on the first day following surgery. For patients who need additional observation, including those whose progress with physical therapy is slower than expected, staying at the hospital for an additional day or two is not uncommon.

A small number of patients may not progress in the hospital as quickly as they would like. This could occur for any number of reasons. In these cases, patients often require additional rehabilitation in skilled nursing or a rehabilitation facilities. Here, trained nursing professionals continue to monitor patients' general health, similar to the hospital setting. Intensive physical therapy

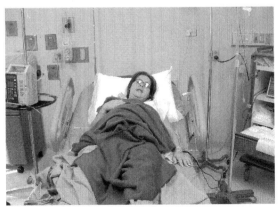

will occur until patients are able to demonstrate their ability to safely and confidently negotiate situations that are similar to the ones they are most likely to experience at home.

There are also certain situations in which it is clear that staying in a skilled nursing or rehabilitation facility will be required, even before a surgery takes place. In the orthopaedic surgeon's office, a social worker or a discharge planner can help make arrangements in advance for assistance at home. A short stay in an extended care facility may also be arranged.

If at all possible, it is best to avoid needing to stay in an extended care facility. Good evidence shows that a patient's chances of returning to the hospital for any number of minor complications is increased if he or she is transferred to one of these settings following hip replacement surgery. It is unclear why this is, but regardless of the reason, being re-admitted to the hospital can be time consuming, costly, and very stressful for patients and their caregivers. (Bernatz, Tueting, and Anderson 2015)

By the time your pain is controlled on a consistent regimen of oral pain medication, you have accomplished your therapy goals (which will be discussed in detail in Section 6: Rehabilitation), and your general health is stable, you should be ready to go home and begin the next phase of recovery. A few aspects of this process that may require special attention include:

Diet

The first aspect of recovery that requires special attention has to do with diet. Diet plays an integral role as patients recover from hip replacement surgery. Recovery from hip replacement requires a tremendous amount of healing to occur, and the body needs nutritional building blocks for this healing to happen correctly. Although there is no clear consensus on which specific diet is best following hip replacement surgery, I recommend that patients aim for a diet that is high in protein, rich in iron, and low in saturated fats, as well as simple carbohydrates.

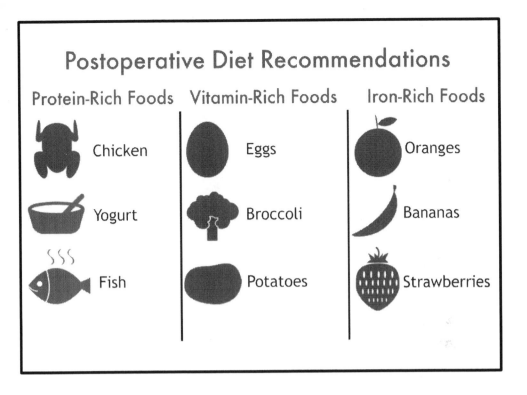

Postoperative Diet Recommendations

Protein-Rich Foods	Vitamin-Rich Foods	Iron-Rich Foods
Chicken	Eggs	Oranges
Yogurt	Broccoli	Bananas
Fish	Potatoes	Strawberries

Poor nutrition leading up to and following hip replacement surgery has been associated with complications. Patients with poor diets have an increased risk of infection following hip replacement.

Your surgeon will likely order laboratory tests to evaluate your nutrition, and depending on the results, he or she may recommend a nutritionist leading up to surgery. (Walls et al. 2015)

Wound Care

Caring for your surgical wound once you return home is another important part of early recovery. A surgeon will likely evaluate your incision prior to leaving the hospital, and you will be instructed on the specifics of how to change your bandage. The following is a general overview of how to care for your wound.

Depending on how long you were in the hospital, you may need to wait a day or two before showering.

Most surgeons will recommend waiting at least 72 hours following surgery before taking a shower. Unless you have been sent home with a waterproof dressing, which you would be instructed on how to use prior to leaving the hospital, you will need to remove your wound dressing before showering. It is generally recommended that you allow soap and water to run over the wound while still avoiding any direct scrubbing or washing. This process is then followed by patting the wound dry and reapplying the dressing.

These guidelines are strictly limited to showering and do not include taking a bath. Specific timing may vary based on your surgeon's preference, but most surgeons will recommend that patients wait at least two weeks before soaking their wounds in a bathtub or swimming pool. This allows the wound time to seal completely and prevents bacteria from accessing the wound.

Once you are safely at home, and your wound is no longer having any areas of drainage, wearing a bandage is a matter of comfort and choice.

Some experts believe it is better to wean from using bandages sooner, rather than later, because this may help the injured skin nerves readjust to the normal sensations of everyday life.

Other surgeons believe that keeping the wound covered until it is completely healed lowers the risk for infection. You will receive specific instruction on this topic prior to leaving the hospital, but be sure to ask your surgical team if you are not sure of your personal surgeon's wound care protocol.

Most patients will return to their surgeon's office two weeks after surgery. At this time, they are evaluated by a member of the surgeon's team for wound healing, pain medication use, blood thinner use, walker or cane use, and therapy progress.

This is generally a very short visit, and increasingly, this can be done remotely with the assistance of a local provider. For patients who live a distance from their surgeon's office, having a remote follow up appointment can save time and decrease travel costs. The possibility for following up remotely should be discussed with your surgeon prior to the date of surgery.

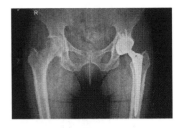

X-rays are a routine method for monitoring hip implants.
You will have x-rays taken after your surgery, while you are in the hospital. You will then have another set of x-rays taken of your new hip replacement approximately six weeks after surgery.

If you have any issues or concerns before your two week follow-up, your surgeon should have a mechanism in place for reaching his or her office and connecting with a staff member who can help navigate the problem. In the event of an emergency, always call 911 or proceed directly to your nearest emergency department. Short of this, your surgeon's office should remain your point of contact.

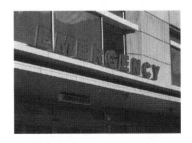

If you have any concerns after being discharged from the hospital, always call your surgeon's office.
You should have clear contact information for your surgeon's team in the event you have any concerns after returning home. If you experience a true emergency, proceed directly to your nearest emergency department and instruct the staff to inform your surgeon immediately,

Now, it may be apparent that relatively little attention has been paid to physical therapy and rehabilitation, which plays a significant role in recovery at the hospital, as well as at home.

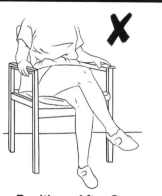

Seating Positions After Surgery
Many natural sitting positions are dangerous following hip replacement. For example, sitting with your legs crossed increases the risk of dislocation, and it should be avoided. The height of your hip joint should be higher than the height of your knee joint whenever you're in a seated position.

We will cover this topic, as well as other aspects of physical therapy and rehabilitation, in much more detail in Section 6: Rehabilitation.

4.1 Precautions

Following hip replacement surgery, there are certain activity and motion precautions which are necessary to minimize the risk for hip joint dislocation. Again, this follows from the idea that in the early period following hip replacement surgery, the patient is fixed, but not yet healed.

Common precautions vary based on the approach used to access the hip joint during surgery. Generally, this is either from the front — as in, a direct anterior or anterior approach — or from the back, which is known as the posterolateral or posterior approach.

The specific approach used for your surgery will be largely based on your surgeon's training and comfort level. Despite the marketing push toward the anterior approach, objective data indicates that there is no difference between the two with regard to overall complication rates, dislocation, recovery, and long term function. What is clear is that you want a surgeon who is comfortable with and experienced at performing the approach that he or she is using. (Lee and Marconi 2015) As we will cover these precautions in detail in Section 6: Rehabilitation, we will only briefly discuss them in this section.

For the anterior approach, a physical therapist will instruct you on how to avoid putting your hip in extended or externally rotated positions. Patients are most likely to find themselves in these positions when they are getting into a car, getting out of a shower or bathtub, or reaching up for something on a tall cabinet. If your surgeon used a posterior approach, then you will want to avoid bending your hip past 90 degrees, bringing your leg inward, or internally rotating your hip.

The most common scenarios for these positions are while rising from a chair or toilet seat, bending down to the floor, or crossing your legs. Several strategies can be used to help remain conscious of your body position, and avoid these "positions of danger," in the weeks following hip replacement surgery. An experienced physical therapist should be able to find the right method for you. We will cover some of the most popular strategies later in Section 6: Rehabilitation.

In terms of activities in the early period following hip replacement, you will largely be limited by your energy level and soreness around the surgical area. This being the case, I recommend that patients limit their activities to walking and climbing stairs, when necessary. Patients should avoid all other physically taxing endeavors.

As your endurance and strength increases, and you gain confidence in your new hip, you may increase the amount and distance that you walk. However, it's still important to be cautious and not to overextend yourself during this first phase of recovery.

Extended Recovery

Congratulations on making it to the six week mark. The most challenging parts of the recovery process should be behind you, and it's likely that you're already walking without a cane or walker.

Most surgeons schedule follow up appointments around the six week point in order to review which pain medications their patients are taking and whether they are still using walking aids to get around. The six week appointment provides a good opportunity to discuss any specific issues or concerns you have with your surgical team, as well.

As a general rule, patients should expect to be off all pain medications and walking without a walker by the six week postoperative appointment.

A full return to daily activities will likely take place around the three month mark, and 95% of the recovery should take place by six months. The final 5% of a patient's recovery occurs between six and 12 months after surgery takes place.

How your personal recovery unfolds largely depends on how debilitated you were prior to your total hip replacement, as well as how active you have been in the early part of your recovery. If you go into surgery with severe pain, already taking

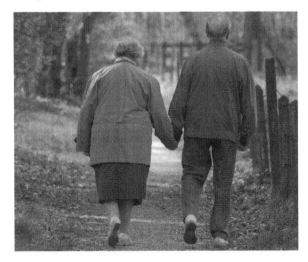

prescription pain medications, and you are unable to do most daily activities, then you may have a longer than average recovery period. It's important to have realistic expectations regarding your recovery from total hip replacement.

Patients who are very active following surgery may also have recovery periods that are atypical. Some of my most energetic patients have had trouble sticking to their post-surgery activity recommendations because they were not in severe pain prior to surgery. What these patients don't realize is that muscles become deconditioned after surgery. This deconditioning, coupled with the injury from the surgery itself, makes the area surrounding the hip very sensitive to activity and prone to inflammation, swelling, and pain. Therefore, patients who consistently push themselves to the limit following surgery may have longer recovery periods.

Depending on how you are feeling at the six week appointment, your surgeon may ask you to return to his or her office again in six more weeks (at the three month mark).

Plenty of successful recoveries do not follow an average timeline, however it is important for your surgeon to track your progress to

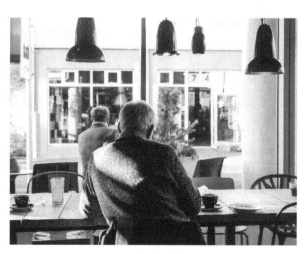

ensure you're continuing to move in the right direction. If that continued progress is not occurring, then it is important to look into why this may be. Early interventions are preferable in order to prevent prolonged pain and disability.

5.1 PRECAUTIONS

Patients are at the greatest risk for dislocation during the first six to eight weeks after surgery. The specific length of time that patients are asked to strictly follow activity and motion precautions following surgery will depend on their surgeon's specific regimen.

At some point—usually between six weeks and three months—your surgeon will tell you it's finally safe to relax somewhat on these activity and motion precautions. It is nearly universal, however, for surgeons to recommend following these precautions whenever possible. I recommend that patients continue to be proactive by staying aware of their body mechanics and positions during both the early and extended recovery phases.

When patients are attuned to their bodies, they are less likely to put themselves in dangerous positions. This means that if you begin to feel discomfort or a sense of danger, regardless of your activity, then you should take a step back and readjust or ask for help.

During the extended phase of recovery you will go through physical therapy and will have the opportunity to discuss many different strategies for minimizing the risk of hip dislocation for the activities specific to your life and based on the unique characteristics of your total hip replacement surgery.

The most common of these will be covered in greater detail in Section 6: Rehabilitation.

Assuming you are feeling healthy and strong at the six week mark, you may be able to skip over the three month follow-up appointment. Instead, you may be asked to return to the surgeon's office at the six month mark. In some cases, surgeons feel confident enough to hold off on seeing patients until the one year mark after surgery. These evaluations may be done remotely, depending on the patient's distance from the surgeon's office. This should be discussed individually with your surgeon.

If at any point there is any issue or concern on your part, your surgeon should have a mechanism for reaching his or her office and connecting with a member of the surgical support team. In the event of an emergency, always call 911 or proceed directly to your nearest emergency department.

Section 6
Rehabilitation

Rehabilitation plays a vital role in recovery following hip replacement surgery. Rehabilitation occurs in phases, which differ in focus and goals. The earliest period of rehabilitation centers on mobility, safety in the home, and strict adherence to motion and activity precautions. Later periods of rehab focus on strengthening the hip and core and increasing activity endurance, as well as safely returning to everyday activities.

Contrary to the common belief, rehabilitation is not only the work of physical therapists. It requires a coordinated effort from orthopaedic surgeons, physical therapists, occupational therapists, case managers, nursing staff, patients, and their families.

Rehabilitation is not limited to the work done following surgery. It really begins the moment you decide to move forward with hip replacement.

Benefits of "Pre-Hab"

Many surgeons are now recommending that patients participate in "pre-hab," which is a preoperative appointment or series of

appointments with physical therapy. Not only will physical therapists offer instructions and preparations for therapy following surgery, but in certain cases, where patients are severely debilitated or deconditioned

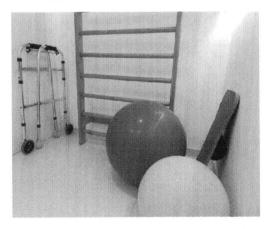

leading into surgery, physical therapists can work on maximizing physical condition before surgery takes place. Good evidence shows that recovery is easier, and potentially more successful, when patients are in better condition heading into surgery. ("Prehab for Surgery" 2016)

During these preoperative evaluations, physical therapists will also discuss modifications to the home and they will make recommendations or provide prescriptions for several medical and non-medical devices that can aid in the early phase of recovery. Some hip replacement centers even have pre-made "Hip Kits," which include several of these devices and implements.

One such kit at the Baptist Health System in San Antonio, Texas, includes a reacher, a long handled shoehorn, a sock donning device, a device to assist in pulling up pants, and a long handled leg washer. This kit also includes guides and recommendations for more permanent modifications that can be made to the home and bathroom.

Patients can easily put together kits of their own using instruments purchased online or at local retailers.

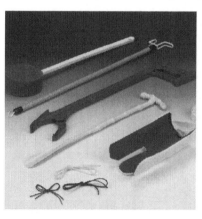

What's In a Hip Kit?
In a study of the most commonly recommended devices, it was found that the top five were:

1) Raised toilet seat
2) Reacher or grabber
3) Abduction pillow
4) Firm seat cushion
5) High chair

(Youm, Maurer, and Stuchin 2005)

Surgery Day

In the hospital, physical therapy typically begins on the same day as surgery. This first therapy session will usually consist of reviewing the precautions for position and motion, followed by sitting on the edge of a hospital bed.

Depending on the discharge plan from your surgeon, this could be the extent of your first therapy session. What is more common, however, is for the therapist to assist you in getting up and ambulating around the hospital hallways or therapy suite.

Post-Op, Day One

On the first day following surgery, most hip replacement patients have two therapy sessions. These sessions pick up wherever the patient left off on day one. Therapists will go over a progressive series of skills and activities necessary for life after hip replacement. These skills may include things like getting into and out of bed, getting to the restroom, sitting and rising from a toilet seat, maneuvering stairs, and getting into and out of a vehicle.

Many hospitals have their own checklists of skills that patients should be able to accomplish and demonstrate safely in order to be cleared for discharge. Once this checklist has been completed, the next phase of therapy and rehabilitation is set to begin.

Not every patient is physically or mentally prepared to return home on the first day after surgery. When this occurs, a serious discussion needs to take place between the surgeon, the patient, and other members of the treatment team.

Based on the patient's need for additional therapy, as well as insurance coverage and personal preferences, there are options for continuing more intensive post hip replacement therapy.

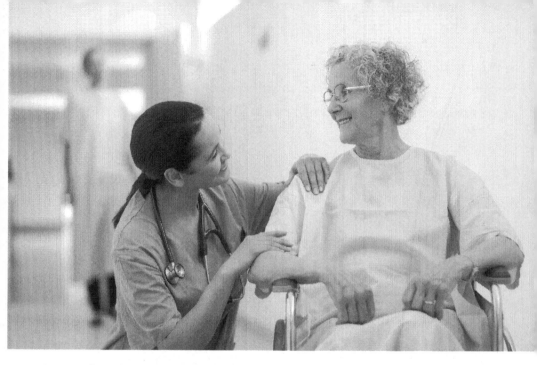

As previously mentioned, this may include a temporary stay at a skilled nursing facility or an inpatient rehabilitation facility. In other cases, it may mean that a patient will be discharged with a home health nurse or therapist.

In each of these scenarios, therapy takes place several times each day. This much therapy is necessary in order to get patients to the point where they can manage life at home and transition to once or twice weekly outpatient therapy, with regular home exercises in between therapy sessions.

Further discussion regarding the differences, benefits, and potential downsides of various rehabilitation options are beyond the scope of this guide. If you believe this may apply to you, please discuss it further with your surgeon.

Outpatient Therapy

After patients return home from the hospital, physical therapy sessions usually take place in the outpatient setting.

These sessions focus primarily on mobility (walking with a walker or cane), navigating the home, and maintaining safe body positions during everyday activities.

Therapists should also be able to demonstrate a few light exercises, which patients will need to continue to work on at home in between sessions. Some therapy clinics offer in-home outpatient therapy, however the availability of these services varies depending on the surgeon and the therapy clinic.

Progress at Six Weeks

Regular outpatient therapy sessions continue once or twice a week for the first six weeks after hip replacement surgery. At that point, most patients return to their surgeons for follow-up appointments, and more custom rehabilitation schedules and plans are often discussed.

By the six week follow up appointment, the majority of patients are ready to progress to a more intensive strengthening program. Weekly outpatient therapy will continue based individual needs and desires.

At this point in the rehabilitation process, a therapist may also recommend activity-specific training and offer advice regarding how to participate safely in recreational sports. Some of the most commonly discussed activities are bicycle riding, skiing, tennis, and golf.

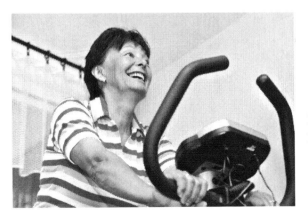

Physical therapy will help you regain strength.
This will occur through safe, everyday activities guided by your physical therapist to ensure you proceed safely.

Activity modifications for these sports will differ based on the approach used during surgery.

As discussed in Section 5: Extended Recovery, personal progress with rehabilitation following hip replacement depends largely on where the patient started from. The general rule for recovery after any orthopaedic surgery, and not just joint replacement surgery, is that patients break muscle down three times faster than they rebuild it. That is to say, if you are inactive for one week, then it will take three more weeks to fully recover. Again, realistic expectations are the key here.

Being too active following surgery can prolong the recovery period and make rehabilitation more difficult. Some common consequences of over-activity are psoas tendinitis, or inflammation of the hip flexor tendon. Another possibility is abductor tendonitis, and trochanteric bursitis, or inflammation of the outside of the hip. And the most significant consequence of over activity is stretching of the healing scar tissue around the hip joint itself, which increases the risk of hip joint dislocation.

This is not to say that patients should not push themselves, or that soreness during rehabilitation isn't to be expected. As the saying goes, "no pain no gain." However, I recommend that patients push themselves to the limit, but never past it.

Precautions During Rehabilitation

Common precautions during the rehabilitation phase after hip replacement surgery fall into two categories.

0 to 12 Weeks Post-Op

During the first 12 weeks after surgery, restrictions in range of motion of the hip are designed to decrease the risk of dislocation.

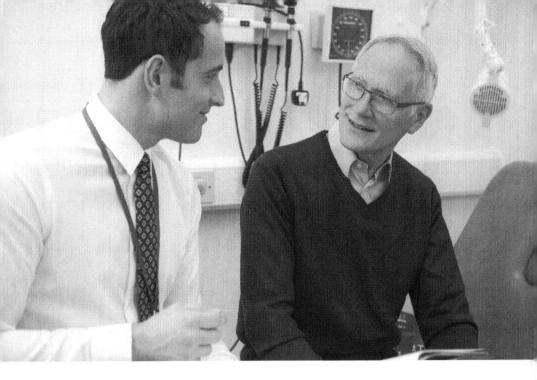

Dislocation of the hip joint is one of the most common reasons why patients need further surgery after total hip replacement. This is a very serious consideration, and it is something most surgeons will keep a close eye on, even though hip dislocation following surgery only occurs in approximately 1% to 2% of cases. (von Knoch et al. 2002)

Restrictions in this early period following surgery are based on the philosophy of being fixed but not yet healed. Regardless of the approach used by the surgeon, direct anterior or posterolateral, surgery has likely weakened the tissues that stabilize the hip. These tissues are commonly repaired in surgery, but they do take time to properly heal.

If patients do not restrict their motion during this early healing period, it is possible to stretch these tissues, or at worst, tear them. Tearing the tissue could cause immediate dislocation or put patients at risk for dislocation in the future.

Reaching the 12-week mark following surgery is a time for celebration.

At this point, the tissue in the hip area has adequately healed and most patients should be ready to go about their daily activities. However, it is still important to be mindful of posture and body mechanics. I recommend that patients always listen to their bodies and avoid putting themselves into uncomfortable or potentially dangerous positions.

The specific positions to avoid during the late phase of rehabilitation will vary based the type of approach used by the orthopaedic surgeon. For the direct anterior approach, it is best to avoid any hip extension beyond neutral, as well as external rotation. The most common reason why patients find themselves in this position is when reaching for an object on the opposite side of the replaced hip or when they are getting into a tall vehicle.

Patients who've had a posterolateral approach will want to avoid flexion beyond 90 degrees, internal rotation of the hip, and adduction of the leg toward the midline.

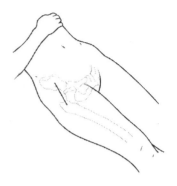

The direct anterior approach accesses the hip from the front
The incision is on the upper-outer aspect of the thigh and ranges from four to eight inches in length.

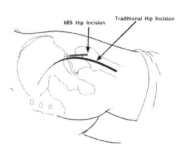

The posterior approach accesses the hip from the back
The incision is on the outer portion of the hip itself and curves toward the buttock. It ranges from four to ten inches in length.

Common sources of dislocation in this manner include rising from a chair or toilet seat and reaching down to pick up an object from the floor.

In either case, significant time will be spent going over these precautions, both during rehabilitation while in the hospital and during subsequent therapy sessions after leaving the hospital.

It can be difficult to follow all of these precautions and avoid putting the body into restricted positions following surgery. Almost every patient has a lapse at some point. However, it is also expected that patients will do their best to adhere to these precautions. Dislocation after hip replacement, while thankfully a rare event, is a big deal and it entails pain, an emergency room visit, anesthesia, and a closed, but possibly open, procedure to relocate the hip.

Once a dislocation occurs, the clock re-sets in terms of following basic precautions and allowing the tissues in the hip adequate time to heal. For a small percentage of patients, dislocation can become a recurrent issue that may require several operations. For all of these reasons, it is important to follow your surgeon's precautions and avoid letting a dislocation happen in the first place.

Section 7
Sports & Exercise

Getting back to normal life after hip replacement surgery means resuming physical activities. However, a certain amount of caution is still needed to prevent hip dislocation. By the time most patients reach the six week mark post-surgery, physical therapists are usually able to start recommending activity-specific training and offering advice on how to participate safely. The specifics of these recommended activity modifications will depend on the type of approach used during the hip replacement surgery.

In my experience, patients tend to be most interested in how they can resume lifestyle sports, such as bicycling, skiing, tennis, and golf. However, because specific activity modifications differ so significantly depending on the approach used during surgery, I recommend that all patients discuss this topic with their surgeons during their post-surgery follow up appointments.

Biking

Bicycle riding is a great, low impact, heart healthy activity following hip replacement surgery. For patients with an anterior approach for

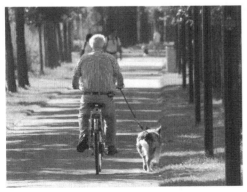

hip replacement, the risk for dislocation primarily occurs while mounting or dismounting the bike. To decrease this risk and maintain good body position, it may be helpful to use some type of step when getting onto the bike, such as a curb.

Patients with the anterior approach for hip replacement will want to avoid extending the hip too much. This can easily happen if the seat is positioned too high. I recommend working with specialists at your local bicycle shop, or adjusting the seat on your own to lower it to a comfortable position that doesn't require too much hip extension. Patients with a posterior approach for hip replacement surgery should avoid deep flexion of the hip. On a bicycle, this occurs during the revolution of the pedals.

The best way to avoid flexion while pedaling is to raise the bicycle seat so that your knees do not go higher than your hip. This may limit the type of bicycle that you can ride, and it will eliminate any competitive road bikes that require a deep lean forward. A local cyclery will be able to offer you a variety of bike options that meet your needs during rehabilitation, while still allowing you to maintain your precautions.

Skiing

Skiing is a popular activity to participate in following hip replacement surgery. Skiing is relatively safe, particularly when it comes to maintaining the proper hip position. However, there are a few exceptions that are important to note before hitting the slopes. The first exception has to do with moguls.

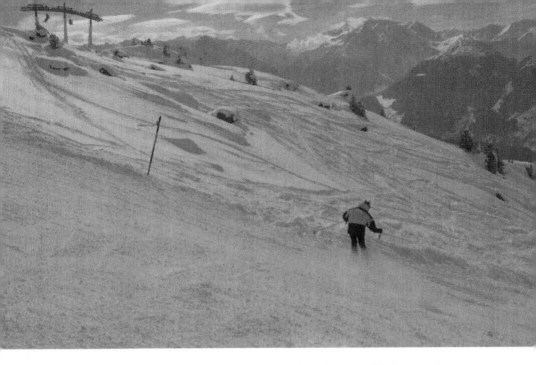

Moguls put significant stress on the hip implant, which can increase the wear rate. Mogul skiing also puts your hip in significant amounts of flexion. I typically recommend that patients not participate in moguls skiing for these reasons.

The second scenario in which you can put yourself into danger on the ski slope is by falling. Of course, nobody plans on falling when they ski. But falls do happen, and for adults who have had hip replacement, falls while skiing can be especially dangerous. You can decrease this risk by sticking to well-groomed runs with mild to moderate difficulty levels. You should also discuss this topic with your physical therapist and surgeon. An experienced therapist will have tips for falling safely or be able to point you to additional resources to help.

Tennis

Tennis is a sport that is difficult on hip replacements. For this reason, it is recommended that singles tennis be avoided entirely following hip replacement surgery.

Doubles tennis and pickleball are okay, given their more strategic nature and relatively limited motion.

The areas where doubles tennis and pickleball put you at increased risk for dislocation are when reaching for out of position shots and when pivoting. While it may be difficult to put yourself in these positions, or let the point go on account of your hip, it becomes very important to think about these scenarios and plan out what you can and will do to avoid putting yourself at risk for dislocation.

Golf

Golf is a wonderful sport to enjoy following hip replacement surgery. In fact, the desire to get back to golfing on a regular basis is a common reason why many people initially consider surgery.

Similar to tennis, the positions of danger in golf occur during the follow through, when pivoting on the replaced hip. This is generally not difficult to work around, but it can sometimes necessitate work with a club pro in order to make swing modifications. Most people can expect to pick up right where they left off before surgery. Few, if any, modifications to a golf swing are necessary, as long as patients continue to be aware of their body position while playing the sport.

It bears mentioning that research has demonstrated that golf handicaps should not be affected by hip replacement surgery. Having knee replacement surgery, on the other hand, will increase your handicap. (Mallon and Callaghan 1992) (Mallon and Callaghan 1993)

The main risk of playing golf after hip replacement has to do with dislocation, and to a lesser extent, wear of the plastic components.

Swing Adjustments

Most patients returning to golf after hip replacement will not need to make significant adjustments to their swings. If, however, a golfer's swing places a high degree of stress on his or her hip, then changes may be necessary.

- *Make sure your clubs are light and flexible. This can reduce strain on your hips and legs throughout your swing.*

- *Opening up your stance may relieve discomfort.*

- *Another common adjustment that golfers make following surgery is to switch to a walk-through or step-through follow through. This may put less strain on your legs and hips.*

- *Decrease the swing plane in the direction of the impacted side to minimize stress on the join.*

PGA champion golfer Gary Player has perfected these techniques, and his strategies can be seen in many online videos.

In terms of dislocation risk, it should be said that there are many people who return to golf after hip replacement surgery, and dislocation is very rare. However, there are things that you can do to minimize the chances of a dislocation occurring.

Starting slow is important. I recommend beginning with partial swings and working up to full swings over time. Work on chipping and putting, and then work toward driving in the later stages of recovery.

Most golfers will use motorized carts for the first year after total hip replacement, even for nine hole outings. It may be wise to continue with a motorized cart, or at least a pull cart, even after the first year of recovery after surgery is complete.

Spike-less shoes are also a good idea, as spikes can transfer significant stress to the hip during the swing and follow through.

Maximizing Results

Everyone who undergoes hip replacement surgery hopes for a successful outcome, but whether or not that goal is met is determined largely by the patient's expectations going into the procedure. From the surgeon's perspective, the fundamental goals of hip replacement surgery include decreased pain, increased function, avoidance of complications, and patient satisfaction. These are not achieved in isolation, and they are all related to varying degrees.

In this section, we will discuss these fundamental goals and some of the ways that you can improve your chances of a successful outcome following hip replacement surgery.

Decreasing hip pain, much like increasing function, depends largely on your starting point. If you have very little pain to begin with, it is unlikely that hip replacement surgery will improve your situation. On the other hand, if you have significant pain that limits everyday functions, then achieving this goal will be relatively easy.

This concept is known as the Delta Effect. If a 20-year-old's hip is the ideal, or 100%, then hip replacement surgery can reliably get older patients to around 80% function. If your current hip status is at 20% function, then getting to 80% is a significant improvement. But, if you are already at 70% function prior to surgery, then the benefit of going through a large operation and difficult recovery process just to get an additional 10% function may not outweigh the risks.

It is a common misconception, even by other physicians, that arthritis on x-rays always warrants joint replacement.

The truth is, arthritis on x-ray does not always correlate with symptoms. If a patient has little pain and he or she is not limited in mobility, then a hip replacement is not the right procedure.

On the other side of this coin is the patient with arthritis that appears mild on x-ray, even though the patient experiences significant pain and functional limitations. It is not uncommon in this scenario for advanced imaging, such as MRI, to shed light on more significant joint damage than is present on x-ray. Therefore, the severity of arthritis that shows up on an x-ray is not the only factor that should be used in determining whether a patient is a suitable candidate for hip replacement surgery.

Self-Managing Pain

Many patients ask what they can do to decrease hip pain on their own. You may think there is very little to be done without surgery, but there are actually many exercises and pain management techniques that have been shown to decrease discomfort leading up to joint replacement surgery and improve pain following surgery, as well.

Pain management is a popular topic within the orthopaedic community. Many physicians are quick to prescribe powerful pain medications, called opioids, to patients leading up to joint replacement surgery, however these medications can have several unintended side effects.

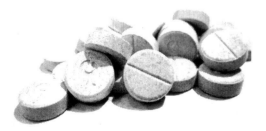

Opioid pain medications are a necessary part of recovery.
To help the medication be as effective as possible after surgery, you should avoid their use before surgery.

Opioid medications may cause constipation, impaired thinking, nausea, and impaired sleep, among many other side effects. The human body can also build up a tolerance to these medications. This tolerance can be harmful, both because of the increased side effects that come with the higher doses of medications needed to achieve the pain-relief effect, and also from the difficulty with pain control following surgery.

Once the body gets accustomed to powerful opioid medications, it is hard to control pain without higher and higher doses, which increases the risk of adverse events.

Taking high doses of opioid medications also slows rehabilitation, putting patients at risk for serious complications such as blood clots, pneumonia, bedsores, and falls.

Taking opioid medications is unavoidable in some situations. In those cases, I recommend going about pain management very carefully and always under the guidance of a primary care provider or a pain management specialist. Whenever a choice is available, patients should always try to avoid using opioid pain medications prior to and following surgery. Avoiding the use of unnecessary opioid medications is one of the smartest things a patient can do to improve his or her chances of a successful outcome following hip replacement surgery.

One way that patients can decrease hip pain without relying on pain medications is by maximizing physical fitness leading up to surgery. As touched on in Section 6: Rehabilitation, "pre-hab" has been shown to make recovery significantly easier and improve long-term outcomes. (Ritterman and Rubin 2013) This serves to increase overall muscle strength and body coordination, both of which are factors that can decrease the forces on arthritic joints and prevent further damage.

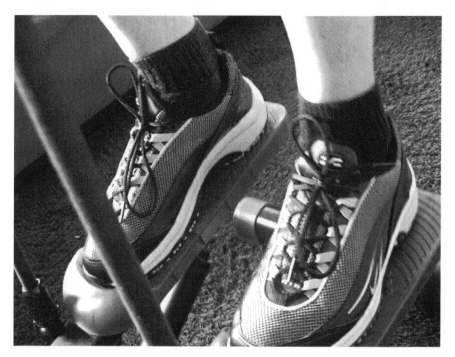

The easiest way to conceptualize this is to think back to a time where you stepped off of a curb without realizing it. The jolt you felt in your joints was the sudden increase in force being applied to them. When your muscles are weak, this happens with every step, though on a much smaller scale. Damage can accumulate rapidly for a person who takes upwards of 5,000 to 10,000 steps each day. Strong muscles are better able to share the load of everyday wear and tear that joints would otherwise bear on their own.

For patients who are looking for natural solutions for pain management, either before hip replacement surgery or in lieu of surgery, I recommend maximizing physical fitness and increasing muscle strength by participating in low impact fitness activities.

Strategies for Avoiding Complications

Another key ingredient to achieving a successful outcome after total hip replacement surgery is avoiding postoperative complications. This is a broad topic that expands beyond the scope of this guide.

However, I believe patients should know that there are things they can personally do to decrease instances of postoperative complications and improve the odds of successful outcomes following surgery. Broadly speaking, the areas where patients can have the most impact have to do with managing diet, vices, and the optimization of other health concerns.

Diet and nutrition are increasingly recognized as important areas for avoiding serious complications following several types of surgery, including hip replacement. (Walls et al. 2015) Serious complications that can result from malnutrition include wound healing issues and infection. Malnutrition can also delay recovery, as it is impossible to build muscle and strength without the adequate nutritional building blocks.

Any number of different diets and strategies can help patients improve their nutrition status leading up to surgery. There are several commonalities among the most successful diet plans. These are frequent small meals, a focus on foods that are high in protein and fiber, staying well hydrated, and avoiding fried foods, fatty meats, and processed foods.

As just one example of this, I have included an informational handout developed in association with the nutrition department at Oregon Health & Science University, in Portland, Oregon, and based upon the "Healthy Eating Plate" from Harvard Medical School and Harvard School of Public Health in Boston, Massachusetts.

Although every patient should take steps to improve his or her nutrition prior to surgery, the specifics of any diet plan should be discussed personally with a surgeon.

Pre-Surgery Diet

Don't skip meals. Eat within one hour of waking, then have a meal or snack every three to four waking hours.

Include lean protein and a high-fiber food (such as fruit, vegetables or a whole grain) at all meals and snacks.

Aim for 64 ounces of fluids daily in order to stay hydrated; choose water or other calorie-free beverages.

Use the "Healthy Eating Plate" below to create balanced, nutritious meals. Avoid fried foods, fatty meats, and processed foods.

Snack ideas:
▶ Greek yogurt & fruit
▶ Small handful of nuts and dried fruit
▶ Hummus and veggies
▶ Low-fat cheese & four whole grain crackers
▶ Peanut butter or almond butter with apple slices

Healthy Eating Plate

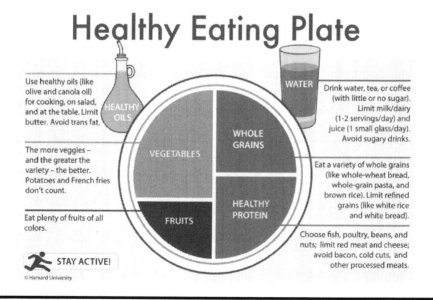

Use healthy oils (like olive and canola oil) for cooking, on salad, and at the table. Limit butter. Avoid trans fat.

The more veggies – and the greater the variety – the better. Potatoes and French fries don't count.

Eat plenty of fruits of all colors.

STAY ACTIVE!

© Harvard University

WATER

Drink water, tea, or coffee (with little or no sugar). Limit milk/dairy (1-2 servings/day) and juice (1 small glass/day). Avoid sugary drinks.

Eat a variety of whole grains (like whole-wheat bread, whole-grain pasta, and brown rice). Limit refined grains (like white rice and white bread).

Choose fish, poultry, beans, and nuts; limit red meat and cheese; avoid bacon, cold cuts, and other processed meats.

Surgeons frequently talk about optimizing general health as a way to minimize the risk of complications following surgery. To a certain degree, this is a general requirement before anyone can qualify for surgery. Most surgeons will require that patients undergo evaluations by their primary medical doctors to assess suitability for surgery.

Patients who already know they have underlying medical issues should take steps to be proactive in getting these health issues in order before moving forward with hip replacement surgery. Doing so can be beneficial, not only because it decreases the risk of complications, but also because it will improve the patient's overall health and well-being.

The most common health issues that are associated with increased risk of complications in and around hip replacement surgery are diabetes, obesity, heart disease, and vascular disease. Again, it is imperative that patients speak with their primary medical doctors about these topics before and after surgery. A primary doctor is the person best equipped to help manage these medical issues on a long-term basis.

Limiting Vices

While not a medical issue, per se, smoking is another area that should be addressed prior to moving forward with hip replacement surgery. Many surgeons have strict rules against smoking, and they will not provide surgery to patients who are current smokers. Some surgeons even go as far as testing their patients' blood for nicotine prior to surgery.

Smoking increases the risk of surgical complications. Specifically, it makes patients prone to experiencing some of the most dangerous complications.

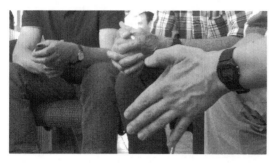

Smoking places a new hip at risk.
Most surgeons now have resources available to help in the long and difficult process of smoking cessation.

Examples of the types of dangerous complications that could occur due to smoking would be infection and impaired bone healing, leading to loosening of the implant. Loosening of the implant can cause the type of chronic pain that requires further revision surgery.

These devastating examples of what can happen when a patient smokes prior to or after surgery are only the tip of the iceberg. Smoking also puts surgical patients at an increased risk for blood clots in the legs, blood clots in the lungs, and pneumonia. Prolonged recovery, rehabilitation, and hospital stays are common among patients who smoke prior to surgery, as well.

Most surgeons now have resources available for smoking cessation, and a growing number are providing nutritional guidance and weight loss assistance to patients. Although the availability of these programs varies from surgeon to surgeon, it's not uncommon for top orthopaedic physicians to require patients to take part in nutritional programs and smoking cessation programs before scheduling surgery. These programs are often a good starting point for maintaining health following hip replacement surgery.

Once a patient has had his or her hip replaced, it is imperative that they do their best to make overall health a priority. Serious complications can occur, even years after hip replacement surgery has taken place, if patients continue smoking or eating poorly.

Realistic Expectations

The final goal of hip replacement surgery that we will focus on is overall satisfaction. Satisfaction after total hip replacement is very complex and individual to each patient. Because of that, it is impossible to truly quantify, although many researchers have tried. Several factors that are out of the control of both the patient and the surgeon play a role in satisfaction following hip replacement surgery. Rather than focusing on the factors that are out of their control, I recommend that patients pay attention to factors that are within their control.

Factors that are within a patient's control are considered the intangibles. Trust, rapport, and a good surgeon-patient relationship all play a role in the outcome of a hip replacement surgery. A surgeon who takes the time to explain things in a way that patients understand can make a big difference in how patients feel and how well they recover following surgery. Surgeons should also have empathy for the position their patients are in, and they should ideally provide information on both surgical and non-surgical options for treating hip pain and arthritis.

Patients who feel like they've been provided with all the information necessary before opting for hip replacement surgery tend to report the highest rates of satisfaction. Surgeons should ideally be guiding their patients through the decision making process, rather than dictating which treatments will be done.

As a surgeon, I want all of my patients to feel confident in their decisions to have hip replacement surgery. I never want patients to feel like they are being rushed or forced into doing something they do not want to or are not ready to do. My hope is that everyone is able to find a surgeon who will take the time to answer all of their questions prior to surgery.

I never want patients to have any lingering doubts about which procedures are happening and why that is. Having hip replacement surgery is a big decision, and it should not be entered into lightly.

Realistic expectations of what life will be like following hip replacement surgery will make a big difference in the perceived success of the procedure. In Section 9: A New Normal, we will go into greater depth about how having a hip replacement will impact various aspects of your life.

In brief, I should note that you will never be 20 years old again. Patients who think that having hip replacement surgery will make them feel like they did in their twenties are setting themselves up for disappointment.

The surgeon's goal for hip replacement is to decrease pain in a significant way, and to allow patients to get back to participating in most everyday activities. Few patients are completely pain free following hip replacement surgery. It is normal to have aches and pains with increased activity. It is not uncommon to hear clicks and pops, and patients who have undergone hip replacement will remain at increased risk for complications, such as broken bones and dislocations around the hip, for years to come. Although these risks drop significantly in the early months following surgery, they never go away completely or return to pre-surgery levels.

Section 9
A New Normal

Most patients only consider hip replacement surgery once they've gotten to the point where hip pain is severe enough to limit their ability to participate in the activities they enjoy. As surgeons, our goal is to relieve that pain and get our patients back to their favorite activities and light recreational sports.

With that being said, the truth is that life after hip replacement will always be different than life before. Even the most active and healthy patients still need to avoid participating in repetitive, high-impact activities following hip replacement surgery. The term "high-impact activities" is often used to describe things like running, singles tennis, basketball, and Zumba. At the heart of this recommendation is the concept that, like tires on a car, the materials in a hip replacement will wear out with time and activity. The more stress patients put on their implants, usually through participating in high-impact sports, the greater the chances that future surgeries will be necessary.

A good example of this is the highly-advertised "30-Year Hip."

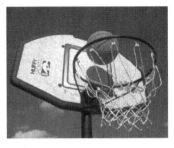

Basketball is not recommended following hip replacement.
If participation in a sport, such as basketball or football, places undue stress on the joint, it's best to become a spectator rather than a participant.

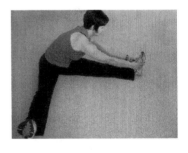

Gentle stretching can make exercise more comfortable.
Low-impact exercise will increase strength and flexibility. Physical therapists can recommend safe stretching techniques after surgery.

The 30-year figure that's often batted around is based on laboratory studies showing that hip prostheses maintain reliable mechanics and function for 45 million simulated walking cycles. If you do the math, over a 30 year span, that averages out to just over 4,100 steps per day. Therefore, the more active patients are following hip replacement surgery, the faster this process will take place and the sooner a second, revision surgery will be required. With any revision surgery, the complexity is greater, and the risks for complications and inferior outcomes increase. As such, surgeons almost always recommend that patients do everything within their control to extend the lifespan of their hip implants.

The risks for complications, such as hip dislocation, bone loosening around the implant, and breaking the bone around the implant, also increase when patients participate in high-impact activities. Thankfully, these complications are rare. This is due in part to restrictions on these sorts of repetitive activities.

In this section, we will focus on what life will be like after hip replacement and the specific activities that are safe to enjoy once the early phases of surgical recovery is complete. There is great variability between physicians and their recommendations for activities that are suitable for adults who have undergone hip replacement surgery. This variability has to do with the art of medicine, the personal experience of the surgeon, and some technical details of each individual procedure. However, there is a general agreement within the orthopaedic community that repetitive, high-impact activity will increase the wear rate of a hip implant and hasten the need for revision surgery.

A study performed in 2009 looked at high-volume hip replacement surgeons and demonstrated the variability in activity recommendations following hip replacement surgery.

"[More than] 95% of the surgeon responses placed no limitations on walking on even surfaces, climbing stairs, bicycling on level surfaces, swimming, and golf for both [total hip replacement] and [total knee replacement]." Following total hip replacement, jogging was discouraged by 71% of the surgeons in this study. Difficult skiing was discouraged by 83%, and singles tennis by 49%.

For total knee replacement, the responses were similar, except the percentage of surgeons who discouraged singles tennis went up to 60%. The occasional game of doubles tennis (one to two times per month) was recommended following total hip replacement by 71% of surgeons. Orthopaedic surgeons who performed a high number of revisions were more liberal in their recommendations to patients, reaching statistical significance for vertical climbing, singles tennis, and bicycling on inclines. None of the surgeons who were surveyed indicated that there was strong scientific evidence for their recommendations. (Swanson, Eli, and Schmalzried 2009)

Returning to Work

The ability to return to work is a high priority for many patients considering hip arthroplasty surgery, especially for younger and more active patients. The length of time that you should expect to be away from work following hip replacement depends on a number of variables, including the demands of your job and the specifics of your procedure.

The guidelines below are rough estimations only:

- Patients with desk jobs will often return to work two to four weeks after undergoing joint replacement surgery. Patients with active occupations may require a longer recovery period.
- Common hurdles to returning to work include postoperative fatigue, swelling, discomfort, and transportation.

Return to work was analyzed in a study of 943 "moderately active" patients under 60 years old who underwent hip arthroplasty surgery. This study found that 90% of young, active patients who were employed before surgery eventually returned to work, with the vast majority returning to their preoperative occupations. Only 2.3% were limited in their ability to return to work because of their operative hip. (Nunley et al. 2011)

Driving a Car

It's not uncommon for patients to be both eager and anxious about driving after surgery, however postoperative medications and restrictions can make driving dangerous during the recovery period. Please consider the following before returning to the road:

The amount of time that is necessary before safely operating a vehicle after surgery varies from patient to patient. Most patients require at least six weeks of recovery following hip replacement before they are ready to drive.

Please use your best judgment in determining when you feel comfortable driving again postoperatively and discuss this further with your surgeon.

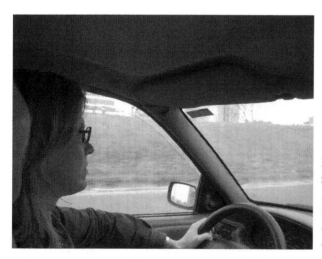

Driving with a hip replacement is safe.
How soon you can return to driving after surgery depends on your progress and comfort.

Do not drive while taking any narcotic pain medications. This is considered driving under the influence.

The reason patients are asked to wait an average of six weeks before returning to the road has to do with reaction times and the ability to perform an emergent stop if the need arises. The research on this issue has been relatively consistent. The traditional threshold has been set at six weeks from the time of surgery before patients can safely drive. More recent research has suggested that with modern accelerated therapy and rehabilitation protocols, up to 87% of patients should be able to return to their pre-surgery brake times by two weeks postoperatively, with remaining patients achieving this level by four weeks postoperatively. (Hernandez et al. 2015)

Another important study looked at return to preoperative brake times based on the hip that was replaced (left versus right). Not surprisingly, this study indicated that patients who had a right hip replacement took significantly longer to return to preoperative brake times than those who had a left hip replacement. In this study, people with right hip replacements returned to preoperative brake times at an average of six weeks following surgery, while those who had a left hip replacement returned to preoperative brake times at an average of eight days after surgery. (Jordan et al. 2014)

Navigating Stairs

Stairs tend to be a trouble area both leading into surgery and immediately following hip replacement.

Prior to leaving the hospital, most patients work with physical therapists on techniques for safely navigating stairs using either a walker, cane, or crutches. This is part of a discharge checklist.

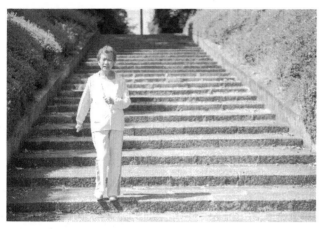

It's not unusual to have trepidation about using stairs after surgery. *Always start with the strong leg when going up stairs and the weak leg when going down.*

However, the techniques recommended by physical therapists usually aren't necessary once the initial recovery phase is complete.

The goal here is for patients to work their way back to going up and down stairs in a tandem fashion, or one leg after the other. This is not easy to recover, especially for people who had trouble on stairs before surgery.

Walking up and down stairs in tandem fashion requires significant muscular strength, which can take some time to regain after surgery.

This weakness can be due to generalized atrophy from decreased activity, or from the approach used in the surgery. In any event, therapists continue to work with patients on these skills for as long as necessary during the early recovery phase.

Climbing Ladders

Ladder climbing is an area of contention amongst joint replacement surgeons. Some orthopaedists recommend avoiding ladders entirely, regardless of whether or not an adult has had hip replacement surgery. Even the most physically fit and coordinated people fall from ladders and can suffer life altering consequences.

As discussed with regard to stairs, climbing up and down ladders requires significant muscular strength. It is likely that the muscles necessary for ladder climbing are weak and atrophied even prior to surgery, which is only made worse by going through a major operation and subsequent rehabilitation.

Only if it is necessary for a patient's occupation would it be recommended to pursue this activity. Even then, it should be cautioned that extreme care needs to be taken when moving up and down a ladder, examples of which include using a spotter or securing the ladder to a structure.

Kneeling & Crawling

Participating in activities that involve kneeling and/or crawling is generally not recommended following hip replacement surgery, as these activities puts the body and hip into unnatural and high-risk positions. The risk here is dislocation, which itself is an extremely unpleasant experience. Dislocated hips require a trip to the emergency room and anesthesia to put the hip back into place. Worse still, a hip dislocation increases a patient's risk of future dislocations.

If kneeling and crawling is required for your occupation, then I recommend discussing the topic further with your orthopaedic surgeon. Otherwise, I would caution against participating in any activities that require kneeling or crawling.

Sex Life

The return to a healthy sex life is one of the less frequently cited benefits of hip replacement surgery. This comes with some caveats, however. Much like yoga and activities that require kneeling or crawling, certain sexual positions can place patients at risk for hip dislocation.

Safe Sexual Positions
Following Hip Replacement

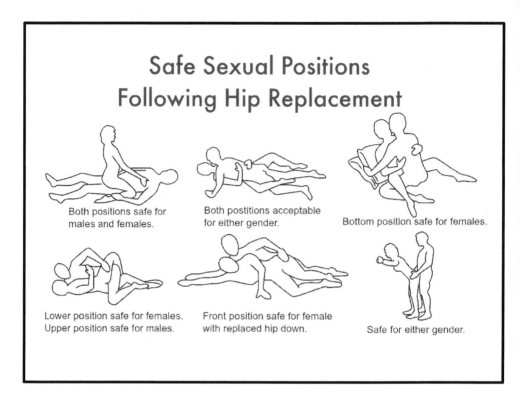

Both positions safe for males and females.

Both postitions acceptable for either gender.

Bottom position safe for females.

Lower position safe for females. Upper position safe for males.

Front position safe for female with replaced hip down.

Safe for either gender.

Simple guides regarding safe sexual positions for men and women following hip replacement surgery are easy to find on the internet. However, some caution should be taken when processing this information. The above diagram illustrates just a few examples of safe positions for both men and women who have undergone hip replacement surgery. Patients should abstain from sex until their surgeons have indicated that it is safe to do so.

The approach used in your hip replacement surgery will influence which sexual positions can be considered safe following surgery. Patients who have had a posterior approach to hip replacement should avoid flexing their hips more than 90 degrees, bringing the leg toward midline, or internally rotating the hip. With hip replacement that's done through the anterior approach, patients should avoid extending the hip beyond neutral, bringing the leg towards midline, or externally rotating the hip.

Travel

Commercial air travel has traditionally been prohibited in the weeks following hip replacement surgery due to a theoretical increased risk of blood clots. While this idea makes sense from a medical standpoint, data on the topic has been mixed, at best. Recent data now suggests that there may be no increased risk for patients who travel by plane in the weeks following surgery. (Cooper, Sanders, and Berger 2014)

Beyond the early recovery phase, there is no increased risk for blood clots during or after flying. It is still recommended, however, that patients get up frequently and move about the aisles, as well as practice calf pumping exercises while seated during the flight. These activities help to maintain blood flow throughout the legs, which may prevent clots from forming.

Continuing Follow Up

Regular follow up with a surgeon is important long after the early recovery phase is complete. This is necessary to ensure that the hip is functioning as it should and that there are no subtle signs of complications with the implant. Every surgeon has his or her own follow up schedule. Some like to see patients every year or two, while others are okay to have their patients come back at five and 10 year intervals following surgery.

After the 10 year mark has passed, it is important to follow up with someone on a yearly or bi-yearly basis. This is necessary to ensure that everything looks good and that the plastic liner within the implant is not wearing out. Even without any symptoms, it is possible a patient may need a small surgery to keep things running smoothly. Waiting until symptoms have begun may require more complex and invasive surgery. Please discuss these expectations with a surgeon.

Other reasons to follow up with a surgeon would be if you have mild pain for more than a week, or anytime you have moderate or severe pain that requires medication. These symptoms could indicate that something is going wrong with the mechanics of your hip replacement hardware, or they may indicate the possibility of an infection.

Section 10
Conclusion

Hip replacement surgery is arguably the most successful surgery ever devised, and if you need to have surgery in 2016, you want it to be a hip replacement. With that being said, surgery is never a walk in the park. Several steps are necessary to make sure hip replacement is a successful procedure.

PREPARING YOUR HOME is very important to set yourself up for success in the early recovery period. There are many potential hazards and dangers in the home that you can identify and mitigate, such as loose rugs and cords. Setting up a recovery center can make your initial time at home easier, as well. Several modifications can be made to the bathroom to make it safe and easy to maneuver following hip replacement surgery.

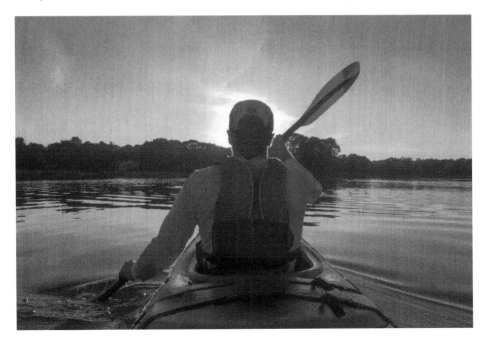

Expect your SURGERY DAY to be very regimented. The details of this day will be covered extensively by your surgeon and at your pre-operative joint replacement classes. Your surgery will roughly take one and a half hours. In most joint replacement centers, you will be up and working with a physical therapist the same day as surgery.

POSTOPERATIVE RECOVERY in the early period following hip replacement surgery is primarily focused on pain management, surgical wound care, and general healing from the surgery. Your pain will be managed using various methods and your general health will be monitored until you are cleared to return home. A physical therapist will also be available to help you master basic daily activities in an efficient and safe manner.

EXTENDED RECOVERY begins after your six week follow up appointment. By this point, you are likely to be feeling much better and you will begin to transition back to your normal activities. While you may feel very close to fully recovered, you will continue to make progress for the first year following hip replacement surgery.

REHABILITATION consists of formal and informal physical therapy. Certain precautions are often necessary in order to avoid complications such as hip dislocation, but with the guidance of a physical therapist, everyday activities can help patients regain strength and build confidence in the weeks and months following surgery.

SPORTS & EXERCISE following hip replacement are typically limited to everyday activities such as walking, hiking, cycling, doubles tennis, and golf.

Specific precautions, and body position techniques, can make it safer to return to the sports and activities you love.

Some of the keys to MAXIMIZING RESULTS following hip replacement surgery include avoiding prescription pain medication, maximizing your physical fitness leading into surgery, and optimizing your general health with the assistance of a primary care provider. Setting realistic expectations can have a significant impact on surgical outcomes. A good relationship and trust with your surgeon goes a long way to helping you establish these expectations, and working together toward a successful hip replacement surgery is always the ultimate goal.

It may take a while to get to A NEW NORMAL, but all hip replacement patients get there eventually. A few considerations should be taken into account to help your hip implant last as long as possible. These boil down to taking care of your hip and your general health, and avoiding activities that put you at risk for falling, dislocation, or excessive wear of your implant. A surgeon can help to monitor the health of your hip and identify problems before they become serious.

Hip replacement surgery can be extremely successful, offering pain relief, increased activity, and return to a joyous life that arthritis prevents many people from living. However, it is also a major surgery with several important drawbacks to consider. Finding a surgeon who you trust, and getting all of your individual questions answered, will help you feel more comfortable moving forward with this life changing surgery.

Section 11
References

For more information on all aspects of total hip replacement surgery, please visit the website for the American Academy of Orthopaedic Surgeons (AAOS). There, you'll find articles, diagrams, and videos describing the entire process.

Below, is a list of references cited within this book.

Bernatz, James T., Jonathan L. Tueting, and Paul A. Anderson. 2015. "Thirty-Day Readmission Rates in Orthopedics: A Systematic Review and Meta-Analysis." PloS One 10 (4): e0123593.

Cooper, H. John, Sheila A. Sanders, and Richard A. Berger. 2014. "Risk of Symptomatic Venous Thromboembolism Associated with Flying in the Early Postoperative Period Following Elective Total Hip and Knee Arthroplasty." The Journal of Arthroplasty 29 (6): 1119–22.

Hernandez, Victor H., Alvin Ong, Fabio Orozco, Anne M. Madden, and Zachary Post. 2015. "When Is It Safe for Patients to Drive after Right Total Hip Arthroplasty?" The Journal of Arthroplasty 30 (4): 627–30.

Horlocker, Terese T., Sandra L. Kopp, Mark W. Pagnano, and James R. Hebl. 2006. "Analgesia for Total Hip and Knee Arthroplasty: A Multimodal Pathway Featuring Peripheral Nerve Block." The Journal of the American Academy of Orthopaedic Surgeons 14 (3): 126–35.

Jordan, Maurice, Ulf Krister Hofmann, Julia Grünwald, Morten Meyer, Saskia Sachsenmaier, Nikolaus Wülker, Torsten Kluba, and Ingmar Ipach. 2014. "Influence of Left- and Right-Side Total Hip Arthroplasty on the Ability to Perform an Emergency Stop While Driving a Car." Archives of Physical Medicine and Rehabilitation 95 (9): 1702–9.

Lee, Gwo-Chin, and Dante Marconi. 2015. "Complications Following Direct Anterior Hip Procedures: Costs to Both Patients and Surgeons." The Journal of Arthroplasty 30 (9 Suppl): 98–101.

Mallon, W. J., and J. J. Callaghan. 1992. "Total Hip Arthroplasty in Active Golfers." The Journal of Arthroplasty 7 Suppl: 339–46.
———. 1993. "Total Knee Arthroplasty in Active Golfers." The Journal of Arthroplasty 8 (3): 299–306.

Nunley, Ryan M., Erin L. Ruh, Qin Zhang, Craig J. Della Valle, C. Anderson Engh Jr, Michael E. Berend, Javad Parvizi, John C. Clohisy, and Robert L. Barrack. 2011. "Do Patients Return to Work after Hip Arthroplasty Surgery." The Journal of Arthroplasty 26 (6 Suppl): 92–98.e1–3.

"Prehab for Surgery." 2016. Arthritis.org. Accessed February 4. http://www.arthritis.org/living-with-arthritis/treatments/joint-surgery/preparing/prehab-surgery.php.

Ritterman, Scott, and Lee E. Rubin. 2013. "Rehabilitation for Total Joint Arthroplasty." Rhode Island Medical Journal 96 (5): 19–22.

Swanson, Eli, Swanson Eli, and Thomas P. Schmalzried. 2009. "Activity Recommendations Following Total Hip and Knee Arthroplasty: A Survey of the American Association for Hip and Knee Surgeons." The Journal of Arthroplasty 24 (2): e37.

"Total Hip Replacement-OrthoInfo - AAOS." 2016. Accessed February 3. http://orthoinfo.aaos.org/topic.cfm?topic=a00377.

von Knoch, Marius, Daniel J. Berry, W. Scott Harmsen, and Bernard F. Morrey. 2002. "Late Dislocation after Total Hip Arthroplasty." The Journal of Bone and Joint Surgery. American Volume 84-A (11): 1949–53.

Walls, Jason D., Daniel Abraham, Charles L. Nelson, Atul F. Kamath, Nabil M. Elkassabany, and Jiabin Liu. 2015. "Hypoalbuminemia More Than Morbid Obesity Is an Independent Predictor of Complications After Total Hip Arthroplasty." The Journal of Arthroplasty 30 (12): 2290–95.

Youm, Thomas, Steven G. Maurer, and Steven A. Stuchin. 2005. "Postoperative Management after Total Hip and Knee Arthroplasty." The Journal of Arthroplasty 20 (3): 322–24.

FAQs

The following is a brief list of frequently asked questions that can help to make you feel more comfortable with the process of undergoing a hip replacement surgery. This is by no means an exhaustive list, and you will likely think of questions that are not present in this list. These, and other questions you may think of, should be further discussed with your surgeon.

Q. HOW LONG WILL MY NEW HIP LAST?

A. We expect most prostheses to last more than 10 to 15 years. However, there is no guarantee and 10% to 15% may not last that long. A second replacement may be necessary beyond this time period.

Q. WHY DO JOINT REPLACEMENTS FAIL?

A. Failures are relatively rare, occurring at approximately 1% per year. The most common reason for failure of a joint replacement is loosening of the artificial surface from the bone. Erosion of the plastic spacer may also result in the need for a new spacer.

Q. WHAT ARE THE MAJOR RISKS?

A. Most surgeries go well, without any complications. Infection and blood clots are the two most common complications. They occur in approximately 1% of cases. To avoid these complications, antibiotics and blood thinners are used.

In addition to special precautions taken in the operating room to reduce the risk of infection, you will also wear anti-blood clotting stockings and perform various exercises to reduce your risk of developing a blood clot. Discuss the specifics with your surgeon.

Q. SHOULD I EXERCISE BEFORE SURGERY?

A. Yes. Prior to surgery, you should either consult an outpatient physical therapist or follow the exercises recommended by your surgeon. Exercises should begin as soon as possible.

Q. WILL I NEED BLOOD?

A. In recent years there has been increasing use of a drug called tranexamic acid (TXA) which has dramatically reduced blood loss and the resulting need for blood transfusion after hip replacement surgery. That being said, transfusions are sometimes necessary. Your blood levels will be checked before surgery and followed after surgery, and only if absolutely necessary will you receive a blood transfusion.

Q. HOW LONG BEFORE I CAN RESUME PHYSICAL ACTIVITIES?

A. You will likely get up with a physical therapist or your nurse the day of surgery. Your activity level will progressively increase as you feel more confident and comfortable.

Q. WHAT IF I LIVE ALONE?

A. It is highly recommended that you arrange for someone to stay with you and provide assistance in the early days and weeks following surgery. It is possible to transfer to a skilled nursing facility for a short while following your hospital stay, but this is not recommended unless absolutely necessary.

Q. HOW LONG DOES THE SURGERY TAKE?

A. Hip replacement surgery takes approximately 60 to 90 minutes to perform. The entire process from the time you enter the operating room, to the time you return to the recovery area will take between two and three hours.

Q. DO I NEED TO BE PUT TO SLEEP FOR SURGERY?

A. It is increasingly common to use a spinal or epidural anesthetic, which numbs the legs and does not produce loss of consciousness. This is coupled with sedation to help you relax during the operation. It is possible that you may choose, or may need general anesthesia (being "put to sleep"). The choice is between you and your anesthesiologist.

Q. WILL THE SURGERY BE PAINFUL?

A. You will have discomfort following the surgery. However, with multimodal pain control techniques, your surgeon and his or her team will keep you as comfortable as possible. Generally, most patients are able to stop using pain medication within one day.

Q. WHO WILL BE PERFORMING THE SURGERY?

A. Your orthopedic surgeon will lead the surgical team during surgery. Many specialists and assistants will contribute to your successful outcome.

Q. WILL I NEED A WALKER?

A. Yes. The length of time you will need this, and if/when you can transition to a cane, or to walking independently, will vary based on your surgeon's protocols and comfort level.

Q. WILL THERE BE ANY SCARRING?

A. Yes. Depending on the approach used for surgery, this can vary widely (anywhere from 4 to 10 inches). There will be some numbness around the scar, which is usually temporary. The scar's appearance will diminish over time, but it will not disappear completely.

Q. WHERE WILL I GO AFTER DISCHARGE FROM THE HOSPITAL?

A. The goal is that each patient is prepared to return to his or her home following discharge. The vast majority of patients are able to go home directly, but some may transfer to a skilled nursing facility or rehabilitation facility.

Your surgeon's and/or the hospital's case manager, in consultation with your surgeon and the rehab team will help you with discharge planning and making the necessary arrangements.

Q. WILL I NEED HELP AT HOME?

A. Yes. During the first several days or weeks after you return home, you will need someone to assist you with meal preparation and personal care. If you go directly home from the hospital, a case manager may arrange for home health care professionals to come to your house if needed. You should make plans to have family or friends available to help.

Preparing ahead of time, before your surgery, can minimize the amount of help needed. Having the laundry done, house cleaned, yard work completed, clean linens put on the bed, and several days worth of single portion frozen meals will reduce the need for extra help.

Q. WILL I NEED PHYSICAL THERAPY AT HOME?

A. Yes. It will be necessary for you to participate in home health or outpatient physical therapy for several weeks following hip replacement. It is generally recommended that you participate in outpatient physical therapy. However, if you are not able to get out easily, then home health therapy may be best for you. Case managers will help you arrange outpatient physical therapy appointments. The length of time required for this type of therapy varies depending on your progress with recovery.

Q. WHEN WILL I BE ABLE TO GET BACK TO WORK?

A. It is recommend that you request at least two months off from work. Most patients can return to work sooner than this, and in doing so, can exceed expectations. Most moderate activity level jobs will require at least four weeks off from work. Less time is needed for jobs which are quite sedentary with minimal mobility requirements. In the hospital, patients are evaluated by occupational therapists who will make recommendations for joint protection and energy conservation on the job. Additionally, accommodations may be needed for you to use a walker at work.

Q. HOW LONG UNTIL I CAN DRIVE?

A. The ability to drive depends on whether surgery was on your right hip or your left hip, and the type of car you have. If the surgery was on your left hip and you have an automatic transmission, you could be driving at two weeks. If the surgery was on your right hip, or if you have a manual (stick-shift) transmission, then your diving could be restricted as long as six weeks. Getting "back to normal" will depend somewhat on your progress. Consult with your surgeon or therapist for advice.

Q. WHEN CAN I HAVE SEXUAL INTERCOURSE?

A. The time it will take to resume sexual intercourse should be discussed with your surgeon.

Q. DO YOU RECOMMEND ANY RESTRICTIONS FOLLOWING THIS SURGERY?

A. Yes. High-impact activities, such as running, singles tennis and basketball, are not recommended. Injury-prone sports, such as downhill skiing can also be dangerous for the new joint.

Q. WHAT RECREATIONAL ACTIVITIES MAY I PARTICIPATE IN AFTER MY RECOVERY IS COMPLETE?

A. You are encouraged to participate in low-impact activities, such as walking, dancing, golf, hiking, swimming, bowling and gardening.

Thank You

Thank you very much for taking the time to read *Life After Hip Replacement: A Complete Guide to Recovery and Rehabilitation.* My hope is that this guide has provided you with a better understanding of what to expect following a hip replacement surgery, and that it will aid you in setting expectations before undergoing total hip replacement. Knowledge is power, and having a complete understanding of all that will be involved in recovering from hip replacement surgery will increase your likelihood of being satisfied during and after the rehabilitation process.

From here, the next step on your journey should be to seek out a qualified surgeon in your local area, based on your own criteria. I also hope you'll visit **www.reddinghipreplacement.com** for more information on orthopaedic developments and trends. Signing up for regular email newsletters is a great way to stay in the loop about all the latest hip replacement techniques.

I also want to take this opportunity to tell you how much work went into creating this guide. This information is the culmination of 27 years of schooling and specialized orthopaedic training. Please do not share this information without prior written consent.

Whether you choose to pursue hip replacement surgery or you decide that you are not yet ready to proceed, I wish for you relief and the ability to return to the activities that you enjoy.

Made in the USA
San Bernardino, CA
03 September 2018